DASH DIET Health Plan

Delicious Recipes to Help Relieve Hypertension

Contents

About the Book

You may have heard of the "DASH diet", learn what delicious foods you can eat to help you lose weight and enjoy great flavors. Get the 411 about the DASH diet and its health benefits in the Introduction. Then get into the good stuff, a collection of recipes for every meal of the day. In the first section, there are appetizer recipes including grilled pineapple, crusty potato skins and lots more. Second, you will find healthy and delicious breakfast recipes like applesauce oatmeal and orange zest waffles. Third are the lunch recipes that are light and delicious. Then, comes the fiery dinner recipes featuring turkey meatloaf, salad and macaroni just to name a few. Lastly, indulge your sweet tooth without even breaking the rules! Enjoy trying this collection of delicious and nutritious DASH diet recipes, while at the same time making new habits.

Introduction

This book includes the delicious and nutritious "DASH diet" recipes. The DASH diet is an acronym for (Dietary Approaches to Stop Hypertension) and are based on clinical studies from 1997 that found that an eating plan which is rich in fruits, vegetables & low-fat dairy foods and lower in saturated fat, total fat & cholesterol, can significantly lower blood pressure. The DASH diet is recommended by the National Heart, Lung and Blood Institute (NHLBI) for lowering blood pressure.

This eating plan is meant for those with elevated blood pressure. It is also a heart-healthy plan that you can easily share with your family. It is rich in magnesium, potassium & calcium, as well as protein and fiber. The DASH diet plan is a well-balanced way of eating which provides a number of choices and is very easy to learn. It focuses on whole foods without chemicals, refining or other processing which is rich in fruits, vegetables & low-fat dairy foods. The diet reduces intake of red meat, fats or sweets. This method has been precisely proven to help people to lose weight, lower blood pressure & cholesterol and even improve mood & cognitive function. In general, the DASH healthy eating plan may also offer protection against osteoporosis, heart disease, cancer, stroke & diabetes. It also helps to reduce the development of kidney stones and risk of developing diabetes. You are giving your body the nutrients it needs, so you will feel great and avoid disease. Best of luck on your journey eating clean and healthy with the DASH diet! These recipes can be a starting point to help you create new favorite meals & healthy living habits.

Disclaimer

Disclaimer and Terms of Use: Effort has been made to ensure that the information in this book is accurate and complete, however, the author and the publisher do not warrant the accuracy of the information, text and graphics contained within the book due to the rapidly changing nature of science, research, known and unknown facts and internet. The Author and the publisher do not hold any responsibility for errors, omissions or contrary interpretation of the subject matter herein. This book is presented solely for motivational and informational purposes only.

Appetizers

Grilled Pineapple

4-8 Servings

1 ripe pineapple (peeled)

1 tbsp. olive oil

1 tsp. ground cinnamon

1/4 tsp. ground cloves

2 tbsp. honey

1 tbsp. fresh lime juice

1 tbsp. lime zest (grated)

1 tbsp. dark rum (optional)

Take a large mixing bowl, add & combine the olive oil with the cinnamon, cloves, honey & lime juice; whisk to blend and set aside. Cut off the poky exterior of the pineapple. Place the peeled pineapple vertical and cut it in half lengthwise. Then cut each half into in to four long wedges and slice away the core. Put the pineapple in the bowl with the mixture & stir well to coat the pineapple. Now, heat a gas grill up and lay the pineapple on the grill. If you don't have a grill, you can place the pineapple on a baking sheet in the oven set to broil. Cook for about 3 to 4 minutes and baste it once or twice with the left over cinnamon mixture. Reduce the heat to low and again baste with the mixture. Grill the pineapple for about 3 more minutes or until the pineapple is tender & golden. Take away the pineapple from the grill & place it on serving plates. Brush it with the rum (optional) & sprinkle with the lime zest. Serve hot and enjoy.

Crusty Potato Skins

2 Servings

2 russet potatoes (rinsed)

2 tbsp. olive oil

1 tbsp. fresh rosemary (minced)

1/8 tsp. freshly ground black pepper

Pre-heat the oven up to 375 degrees. Put the potatoes in the oven & bake them for about 1 hour or until the skins becomes crusty. Then take out and cut the potatoes in half & scoop out the pulp, ensuring to leave about 1/8 inch of the potatoes' flesh attached to the skin. Set aside the pulp for another use. Now, drizzle each potato skin inside with the olive oil. Smash in the rosemary & pepper. Lastly, return the skins into the oven for about 5 to 10 minutes. Then take them out and serve immediately.

Chipotle Flavored Shrimp

4 Servings

1/2 lb. uncooked shrimp (peeled & deveined)

2 tbsp. tomato paste

1½ tsp. water

1/2 tsp. extra virgin olive oil

1/2 tsp. garlic (minced)

1/2 tsp. chipotle chili powder

1/2 tsp. fresh oregano (chopped)

First of all, rinse the shrimp in cold water, pat to dry with a paper towel & set aside. Then make the marinade in a small bowl by whisking together the tomato paste, water & oil. Stir in garlic, chili powder & oregano, mix well. Now, coat the shrimp on both sides with the marinade until thick. Then put it in the refrigerator for an hour or two. Heat up a gas grill or broiler and lightly coat the grill rack or broiler pan with some cooking spray. Place the cooking rack 4 to 6 inches away from the heat source. Place the shrimp on skewers & then onto the grill. Turn over the shrimp every 3 to 4 minutes. Cook until the shrimp are no longer pink; Serve immediately while they are hot.

Sweet & Spicy Snack Mix

12 Servings

30 oz. garbanzo beans (rinsed, drained & pat to dry)

2 c. Whole wheat cereal

1 c. pineapple chunks (dried)

1 c. raisins

2 tbsp. honey

2 tbsp. Worcester sauce (reduced sodium)

1 tsp. garlic powder

1/2 tsp. chili powder

Olive oil

Pre-heat the oven up to 350 degrees. Evenly coat a 15 ½ x 10 ½ inch baking sheet with olive oil. Then, take a heavy skillet and drop a splash of olive oil onto it. Add garbanzos into the skillet & sauté on medium heat for about 10 minutes, stir frequently until the beans start to brown. Take them out and transfer them to the prepared baking sheet. Place in the oven and bake for about 20 minutes, until the beans becomes crispy, stir frequently. Now, lightly coat a roasting pan with oil. Add the cereal, pineapple & raisins into the pan. Stir in the roasted garbanzos, mix evenly. Next, in a large pot add & combine honey, Worcester sauce & spices, stir lightly to mix well. Pour this mixture over the snack mix & toss. Place in oven and bake for about 10 to 15 minutes, stirring occasionally to keep it from burning. Take it out from the oven and let it cool. Serve or store in a sealed container.

Pickled Asparagus

6 Servings

3 c. fresh asparagus (trimmed)

1/4 c. pearl onions

1/4 c. white wine vinegar

1/4 c. cider vinegar

1 sprig fresh dill

1 c. water

2 whole cloves

3 garlic cloves (whole)

8 black peppercorns (whole)

1/4 tsp. red pepper flakes

6 coriander seeds (whole)

Mason jars

First of all, remove the woody ends of the asparagus & cut them to fit into the jars. Place the asparagus in a strainer, wash well & drain. Trim and slice the onions. Combine all ingredients in airtight containers. Serve immediately or store in refrigerator for up to 4 weeks.

Breakfast

Applesauce Oatmeal

2 Servings

2 c. water (filtered)

1 c. oats (unsalted)

1/2 c. golden raisins or cranberry raisins

1/2 c. homemade applesauce

1/2 tsp. cinnamon

Dried cranberries (optional)

1/2 c. orange juice (for 1/2 c. water)

Take a medium sized saucepan; add 2 cups of water and bring it to a boil. Then add in raisins & apple sauce. Keep it boiling; add in the unsalted oats and cinnamon. Remember, you can add more cinnamon if required. Then reduce the heat to medium & stir for 1 minute more. Take away from the heat, cover and set aside for about 3 to 5 minutes. Serve hot and enjoy! You can also use dried cranberries and 1/2 cup of orange juice in-place of half cup of water for a citrusy flavor.

Orange Zest Waffles

4 Servings

For waffles:

1 c. whole-wheat flour

1/2 tsp. vanilla extract

1/3 tsp. ground cinnamon

1 large egg (separated)

1 c. orange juice

1 tbsp. orange zest

1/4 tsp. cream of tartar

1 tsp. baking powder

1/4 tsp. raw sugar

For topping

1 c. homemade applesauce

1 orange (juiced)

Pre-heat the oven up to 350 degrees. Take a large mixing bowl; sift the whole wheat flour & cinnamon together. Then separate the egg (save whites). Add the egg yolk, orange zest, orange juice, baking powder, sugar & vanilla extract into the bowl. Whisk well to make a smooth batter. Now, in a small bowl; beat the egg white and cream of tartar until stiff peaks forms. Fold it into the batter. Then, lightly spray oil on the waffle maker and place 1/2 cup to 3/4 cup of batter on the waffle iron, as required. Bake them in the oven until ready. *For preparing the topping;* in a small skillet add and combine homemade applesauce & the juice of one orange. Cook over low heat and stir occasionally. Serve waffles with topping and enjoy.

Papaya & Coconut Breakfast Shake

2 Servings

1 ripe papaya (seeded, peeled & cut into 1 inch chunks)

1 c. plain yogurt (low-fat)

1 c. coconut water

2 tbsp. wheat germ

Take a food processor or blender, add and blend all the ingredients well. Pour mixture into two serving glasses and enjoy.

Kale & Apple Smoothie

1 Serving

1 c. kale leaves

1/2 sweet apple (cored & coarsely chopped)

1/3 c. apple cider

2 tbsp. sunflower seeds (unsalted)

6 ice cubes

8 fresh mint leaves

Take a food processor or blender, add and puree all the ingredients together well. Pour the mixture into a serving glass & drink while fresh.

Cornmeal Waffles with Blueberries & Yogurt

8 Servings

1 c. whole-wheat flour

1 c. yellow cornmeal

2 tbsp. sugar

1½ tsp. baking powder

1¾ c. low fat milk (1%)

1 tbsp. unsalted butter (melted)

2 tbsp. canola or corn oil

2 large egg whites

2 c. plain low-fat yogurt (for serving)

2 ⅔ c. blueberries (for serving)

Pre-heat the oven up to 200 degrees. Spray a non-stick waffle iron with oil and heat it well. Take a large bowl; add & combine flour, yellow cornmeal, baking powder and sugar; mix them well. Then in another small bowl; whisk together the milk, melted butter and 1 tbsp. of oil. Pour it into large bowl and stir it until it just barely combines (don't over mix). Now, in a medium bowl; beat the egg whites until stiff and fold them into the batter. Pour about 1 cup of batter into the waffle iron, close and cook until waffle is golden browned. Remove the waffles and place on the baking sheet in the oven to keep them warm and toasty. Do the same process for the remaining waffles. Lastly, slice the waffles into squares, top them with 1/4 cup of yogurt & 1/3 cup of blueberries and serve immediately.

Cornbread Recipe

5-10 Servings

1 c. cornmeal

1 c. whole-wheat flour

1/4 c. sugar

1 tsp. baking powder

1 c. low fat (1%) buttermilk

1 egg (whole)

1/4 c. margarine

1 tsp. vegetable oil (for greasing baking pan)

Pre-heat the oven up to 350 degrees. Lightly grease an 8 x 8 inches baking dish. Take a bowl, add & mix cornmeal, flour, sugar & baking powder together. Then, in another bowl, combine buttermilk & egg, beat lightly. Gradually, add buttermilk, egg mixture & margarine into the dry ingredients, mix well. Put the mixture into baking dish and place in oven. Bake it for 20 to 25 minutes. Remove and let it cool. Slice it into 10 squares pieces and serve.

Lunch

Blackened Chicken with Berry Salad

2-4 Servings

4 oz. chicken breast (boneless & skinless)

1 tsp. blackening spice mixture (unsalted)

1 c. romaine lettuce

Grated vegetables e.g. carrots, radishes, tomato, peas etc. (optional)

Berries (optional)

Oil & vinegar or raspberry dressing (to taste)

First of all rub the chicken breast with the spice mixture and grill it until the internal temperature is 165 degrees. Then make the salad base with romaine lettuce strips and top them with vegetables of your choice like grated carrots, radishes, pea pods, red cabbage, tomato and peas etc. Next, top it with a mix of berries; including raspberries, blueberries and sliced strawberries. Then slice the grilled chicken breast into strips & lay them on top of the salad. Top it with your favorite oil & vinegar or raspberry vinaigrette dressing and enjoy. Remember, to check for low sodium on the dressing you choose.

Spicy Seared Fish

2-4 Servings

1 lb. salmon fillet (or any other fish)

1 tbsp. olive oil

1 tsp. spicy seasoning (salt-free)

Pre-heat the oven up to 350 degrees. Rinse and pat the fish dry and place in a dish. Coat a casserole dish with cooking oil spray. Combine oil & seasoning, drizzle it over the fish. Place in oven and bake uncovered for about 15 minutes or until fish flakes with fork. Take out & slice it into four parts, serve with rice.

Marvelous Frittata

6 Servings

6 eggs

1 c. sweet corn (frozen)

1 c. pepper strips (sliced)

1 c. tomatoes (cut in half)

1/4 c. onion (sliced)

2 tbsp. canola oil or coconut oil

1 tbsp. fresh basil (diced)

4 oz. cheddar cheese or other similar (low-fat)

Take a non-stick frying pan; add a splash of oil and warm it on medium heat. Add pepper strips, onion & frozen sweet corn. Cook the mixture for 3 minutes and keep stirring it frequently. Then add in tomatoes, sauté for about 5 minutes or until the onion is translucent, stir continuously. In a small bowl, add eggs and diced basil, mix well. Pour the egg & basil mixture over the vegetables. Lift the edges or divide a little in the center to allow the eggs fall into bottom of mixture while the frittata cooks. Once the egg mixture gets thick then, top it with cheese. Lastly, place under the broiler or grill for 2 to 3 minutes until browned and serve.

Chicken & Spanish Rice

5 Servings

1 c. onions (chopped)

3/4 c. sweet green peppers

2 tsp. vegetable oil

1 c. tomato sauce

1 tsp. parsley (chopped)

1/4 tsp. black pepper

1½ tsp. garlic (minced)

5 c. brown rice (cooked in unsalted water)

3 ¼ c. skinless & boneless chicken breast (cooked & diced)

Take a large skillet; add oil, onions & green peppers. Cook it on medium heat for about 5 minutes. Stir in tomato sauce & spices, heat through. Then add cooked rice & chicken, sauté well until ready. Place in serving plates and enjoy.

Chicken Burritos

4 Servings

For the sauce

1 tsp. oil

1 red bell pepper (chopped)

1 jalapeno pepper (chopped)

2 ribs celery (chopped)

1 yellow onion (chopped)

2 tbsp. cumin seeds

16 oz. grape tomatoes

2 tbsp. fresh oregano

2 garlic cloves (chopped)

8 oz. pre-cooked chicken breast meat

4 whole wheat tortillas

1/2 c. reduced-fat cheddar cheese (shredded)

2 c. green cabbage (shredded)

Take a large skillet; add oil and warm on medium-high heat. Add peppers, celery, onion & cumin, sauté for about 10 to 15 minutes or until lightly browned. Stir in tomatoes, oregano & garlic; cook again for about 5 to 10 minutes. Now, put it to a blender & puree until desired consistency. Next, divide the chicken evenly and place it in the tortillas. Top with cheese, cabbage & sauce. Roll up, serve and enjoy.

Steamed Salmon (Asian-Style)

4 Servings

1 c. chicken broth (low-sodium)

1/2 c. mushroom caps (shiitake) slice

2 tbsp. ginger (mince)

1/4 c. green onions (slice)

1 tbsp. soy sauce (lite sodium)

12 oz. fish fillet (salmon)

Take a large shallow saucepan; add and combine the broth, mushrooms, ginger, green onions and soy sauce. Bring it to a boil on high heat, after it boils lower the heat & simmer for a few minutes. Add the salmon fillets, cover with lid and cook gently for 5 minutes over low heat so that the salmon is flaky. Present on a serving plate and serve one piece of salmon with about 1/4 c. of the broth.

Dinner

Turkey Meatloaf

5 Servings

1 lb. lean ground turkey

1/2 c. regular oats (dry)

1 large egg (whole)

1 tbsp. onion (dry chips)

1/4 c. ketchup (low sodium)

Pre-heat the oven up to 350 degrees. Then, take an oven friendly pan (loaf pan), add & combine all ingredients, mix well. Place in oven and bake for 25 minutes or until internal temperature of 165 degrees. Remove and cut into five slices, serve warm.

Potato Salad

5 Servings

5 c. small potatoes

2 tbsp. olive oil

1/4 c. green onions (chopped)

1/4 tsp. black pepper

1 tsp. dill weed (dried)

First of all, rinse the potatoes. In a saucepan, add the potatoes and boil for 20 minutes or until tender. Take out the potatoes and cool for about 20 minutes. Then, cut them into quarters, stir in olive oil, onions & spices. Place in refrigerator until ready to serve.

Baked Macaroni

6 Servings

1/2 lb. ground beef (lean)

1/2 c. yellow onion (diced)

7 oz. whole wheat elbow macaroni

15 oz. spaghetti sauce (low sodium)

6 tbsp. parmesan low sodium/ reduced fat

Pre-heat the oven up to 350. Heat up a large frying pan and saute the onions with the beef until cooked thoroughly. Next, drain out all of the beef fat and set it aside. Then heat a large pot filled with water over high heat until boiling. Then add in the pasta and cook until tender. Drain the water out and add the noodles to the beef along with the sauce. heat evenly then serve.

Beef & Veggies Kebabs

2 Servings

1/2 c. brown rice

2 c. water

4 oz. lean top sirloin (optional)

3 tbsp. fat-free Italian dressing (low sodium)

1 green pepper (seeded & cut into 4 pieces)

4 cherry tomatoes

1 small onion (cut into 4 wedges)

2 metal or wooden skewers (soak in water for 30 minutes in case of wooden)

Take a saucepan; add water & rice, bring it to boil over high heat. Then, reduce the heat to low, cover & simmer for about 30 to 45 minutes or until rice is tender. If necessary, use more water to keep the rice from drying out. Remove and transfer to a small bowl, keep warm. Now, slice the meat into 4 even pieces. Place the meat into a small bowl and top with Italian dressing. Place it into the refrigerator for about 20 minutes to marinate. Next, heat a gas grill or broiler. Lightly coat the broiler pan or grill rack with cooking spray. Place the cooking rack 4 to 6 inches away from the heat. Thread meat cubes, green pepper slices, cherry tomatoes & onion wedges (2 each) onto every skewer. Place the kebabs on the grill rack or broiler pan and grill or broil the kebabs for about 5 to 10 minutes, keep turning as required. Remove and place on the serving plates and serve with the rice.

Halibut with Tomato Basil Salsa

4 Servings

4 (4 oz. each) halibut fillets

2 tomatoes (diced)

2 tbsp. fresh basil (chopped)

1 tbsp. garlic (minced)

1 tsp. fresh oregano (chopped)

2 tsp. extra virgin olive oil

Pre-heat the oven up to 350 degrees. Evenly coat a 9 x 13 inch baking pan with cooking oil spray. Take a small bowl; add & combine the tomato, basil, garlic & oregano. Then, add the olive oil & mix well. Place the halibut fillets into the baking pan and spoon the tomato mixture over the fish. Place it in the oven & bake for about 10 to 15 minutes or until the fish is opaque throughout. Remove & transfer it to serving plates, serve right away.

Chicken Salad

5 Servings

3¼ c. chicken (skinless)

1/4 c. celery (chopped)

1 tbsp. lemon juice

1/2 tsp. onion powder

3 tbsp. light mayo or miracle whip

First of all; bake the chicken, slice into cubes and refrigerate. Then, in a mixing bowl, add and combine all the other ingredients. When well combined, add the chilled chicken and mix well. Serve cold on whole wheat bread.

Creamy Asparagus Soup

6 Servings

2 c. potatoes (peeled & diced)

1/2 lb. fresh asparagus (cut into 1/4 inch pieces)

1/2 c. onion (chopped)

2 stalks celery (chopped)

4 c. water

2 tbsp. butter (unsalted)

1/2 c. whole-wheat flour

1½ c. fat-free milk

Lemon zest (to taste)

Cracked black pepper (to taste)

Take a large saucepan; add & combine the potatoes, asparagus, onions, celery and water. Sauté over high heat until boiled. Reduce the heat to low, cover & simmer for about 15 minutes or until the vegetables are tender. Melt in the butter. Then in a small bowl, whisk the flour & milk together. Gradually, pour the mixture into the saucepan, stirring frequently. Put the heat to medium high & keep on stirring for about 5 minutes or until the soup gets thick. Take away from the heat and pour it in the soup pot. Season it with lemon zest & cracked black pepper (to taste). Serve it warm and enjoy.

Desserts

Scorched Apples Stuffed with Walnuts & Cranberries

4 Servings

4 apples

1/3 c. walnuts (chopped)

1/3 c. cranberries (dried)

1/4 tsp. cinnamon (ground)

1/4 tsp. nutmeg (freshly grated)

6 tbsp. maple syrup (grade 'B')

1 c. water (boiled)

2 tsp. unsalted butter

1/2 lemon

Pre-heat the oven up to 350 degrees. Cut off the top of each apple to make a lid. Scoop out the core until only 1/2 inch from the apple bottom remains. Then, take a medium bowl; add and mix walnuts, cranberries, cinnamon, nutmeg and 2 tbsp. of maple syrup. Stuff the apples with the mixture and top each with 1/2 tsp. of butter, replace the apple lids. Transfer them to a baking dish and squeeze the lemon juice over the apples. Pour in the boiled water and cover tightly with aluminum foil. Place in oven and bake for 20 minutes. Then uncover and baste with the liquid in the dish. Keep on baking for about 20 to 30 minutes or until apples are tender. Take out and let stand for 5 to 8 minutes. Place each apple into a dessert bowl and drizzle each with 1 tbsp. of maple syrup; serve warm and enjoy.

Buttermilk Soufflés with Fresh Berries

6 Servings

3 tsp. gelatin powder (unflavored)

1/4 c. + 2 tbsp. low fat milk (1%)

2¾ c. buttermilk

1/2 c. honey

1/2 tsp. vanilla extract

Canola oil (for spray)

1/2 c. fresh blueberries

1/2 c. fresh raspberries

Take a small heat proof bowl, sprinkle the gelatin on the milk and let it stand for 5 minutes or until the gelatin absorbs the milk. Then, in a small skillet; add some water and bring to boil over low heat. Place the gelatin mixture bowl into the water for 2 minutes or until gelatin is completely melted & dissolved, stir constantly. Now, in medium sized saucepan, add buttermilk and warm it over medium heat, stir constantly. Remove from heat and stir in the gelatin mixture, mix well until combined. Whisk in the honey and vanilla extract and transfer it to a large measuring pot. Coat ramekins or custard cups with oil and pour buttermilk mixture into them. Cover each with plastic wrap and place in refrigerator for at least 4 hours or until chilled and set. Remove and place on serving plates, sprinkle with blueberries & raspberries and serve chilled.

Cantaloupe & Mint Ice Pops

8 Servings

3 c. ripe cantaloupe (peeled, seeded & cubed)

1/2 c. amber agave nectar or honey

2 tbsp. fresh lemon juice

1 tbsp. fresh mint (finely chopped)

Take a food processor or blender, puree 2 ½ cups of cantaloupe cubes and transfer to a bowl. Finely chop the remaining 1/2 cup of cantaloupe and add to the puree bowl. Add in agave, lemon juice and mint, whisk well. Now, prepare eight ice pop molds and divide the puree among them, cover with lid. Place in the refrigerator to freeze for about 4 hours or until the pops are firm. For serving, take out and rinse the pop mold under lukewarm water. Remove the pop from the mold and serve.

Cantaloupe & Mint Slush

8 Servings

3 c. ripe cantaloupe (peeled, seeded & cubed)

1/2 c. amber agave nectar or honey

2 tbsp. fresh lemon juice

1 tbsp. fresh mint (finely chopped)

First of all; place a metal baking dish or cake pan & a metal fork in the freezer for about 15 to 20 minutes or until well chilled. Then take a food processor or blender, puree cantaloupe cubes. Add in agave and lemon juice and mint, pulse to combine well. Pour this into a disk or pan and freeze for 1 hour or until mixture is icy. Take out and stir the icy crystals into the center by using the cold fork. Place again to freeze for 1 to 2 hours, remove and stir well. Freeze once more for about 4 hours. Take out and serve chilled in bowls immediately.

Fresh Strawberries with Chocolate Dip

4 Servings

1/2 c. low fat (2%) canned milk (evaporated)

5 oz. bittersweet chocolate (finely chopped)

24 strawberries (un-hulled)

Take a small saucepan; add evaporated milk and bring to simmer on medium heat. Remove from heat and add chocolate. Let it stand for about 3 minutes or until chocolate becomes soft. Then whisk well until smooth. Now, divide the chocolate mixture among four small ramekins. Lastly, serve the strawberries with chocolate mixture for dipping and enjoy.

Vanilla Stewed Peaches

4 Servings

1 c. water

1/2 c. sugar

1 vanilla bean (split & scraped)

4 large peaches (pitted & quartered)

Mint leaves or cinnamon (for garnish)

Take a saucepan; add water, sugar, vanilla beans & peaches and warm over low heat. Stir the mixture until the sugar dissolves. Keep on simmering for about 10 minutes or until the mixture is thick. Add the sliced fruit & simmer over low heat for about 5 minutes. Remove and place the peaches & sauce into small serving bowls. Garnish bowls with mint leaves or sprinkle cinnamon. Serve immediately and enjoy.

Peach Crumble

8 Servings

8 ripe peaches (peeled, pitted & sliced)

1 lemon juice

1/3 tsp. ground cinnamon

1/4 tsp. ground nutmeg

1/2 c. whole wheat flour

1/4 c. packed dark brown sugar

2 tbsp. trans-free margarine (sliced)

1/4 c. quick cooking oats (unsalted)

Cooking oil (for spraying)

Pre-heat the oven up to 375 degrees. Coat a 9 inch pie pan with cooking oil lightly. Place peach slices into a prepared pie plate and sprinkle with lemon juice, cinnamon & nutmeg. Then in a small bowl, add and whisk the flour and brown sugar together. Add the margarine into the flour sugar mixture. Add the oats, stir to mix evenly. Sprinkle the flour mixture over the peaches. Place the pan into the oven and bake for about 30 minutes or until peaches are soft and topping is browned. Remove and cut into 8 even slices and serve warm.